Overcoming Erectile Dysfunction

A GUIDE ON UNDERSTANDING ED, EFFECTIVE NATURAL AND HERBAL SOLUTIONS, VITAMINS AND ESSENTIAL OILS FOR ED AND SOME NATURAL VIAGRA

By

Dr. Adam Wells

Copyright

Disclaimer Notice:

Note that it is important that the following information contained in this book is for educational purposes only. After carrying out enough research work, we present a piece of detailed and accurate information as it relates to the present norm. We got the contents in this book from various sources, and hence, the intending readers are not given a warranty. We advise readers to talk to their licensed doctors before trying out the techniques given within this book.

By consenting to this document, the reader accepts that the author is not responsible for any loss either directly or indirectly that can be incurred as a result of the information contained within this book, and also the omissions, errors, or inadequacies of the reader.

Table of Contents

INTRODUCTION

Erectile dysfunction is a condition where a male is unable to achieve an erection or sustain an erection to perform sexual activity. An erection is achieved when the brain sends a chemical signal to the penile muscles causing it to relax. It starts with sexual stimulation that can either be in tactile or mental form. A chemical called nitric oxide released in the nerves is responsible causing the penile muscles to relax and allow rapid blood flow. This blood accumulation fills up the penis much like an inflated balloon and causes it to be erect. When another chemical phosphodiesterase type 5 presents itself, the nitric oxide is broken down causing the penile muscles to constrict again and lose the erection.

It refers to the inability of a male to sustain erection consistently and repeatedly. It is a common problem and is reported that it affects around 18-30 million men. It exerts considerable effects on the quality of life. Most of the time people are reluctant to talk about it to others even to doctors. This is why it is important to address this problem openly.

Erectile dysfunction may include a total and permanent lack of erection, or be a temporary state only. The reasons for erectile dysfunction are many, and therefore there is no universal treatment that helps in all cases. For instance, for older men erectile dysfunction can have physical origins (diseases, injury, etc.) in addition to psychological ones.

Among the many diseases that strike men, one is very special because it strikes not only the body but the soul. Although there are many other much more dangerous diseases, some of them even lethal, erectile dysfunction is a delicate matter because it affects the intimate life of a man. Erectile dysfunction includes multiple sexual disorders, but most often it is considered to be the persistent inability to have an erection or to maintain it for a sufficient amount of time. Erectile dysfunction is often called impotence though this is not precise, because impotence includes other symptoms, like the absence of sexual desire or ejaculation difficulties.

The good news is that at any age, erectile dysfunction is treatable, and very often it is possible to achieve complete recovery of one's sexual powers. It is also encouraging that more men, who have had erectile dysfunction at some time in their lives, admit the presence of the problem and take a proactive approach to discovering the causes and treating them.

On the other hand, even the best treatment cannot substitute for prevention. There are known factors that increase the risk of erectile dysfunction -- tobacco, alcohol, stress, lack of sleep and exercise, anxiety and depression, omission of periodic prophylactic checkups, etc. So even if you trust that modern medical science can help you with erectile dysfunction, do your best to prevent it now, rather than treat it later. As far as recorded history is read, there has been erectile dysfunction in men. In ancient times there were no prescription drugs or psychotherapy in order to help cure the disorder. Many of the ancient civilizations tried to solve erectile dysfunction with a number of different remedies. Many of these remedies are dangerous and harmful to your body, which is why we strongly recommend that you do not use them. Nonetheless, it is interesting to see that ancient peoples dealt with erectile dysfunction just like millions of people to this day.

UNDERSTANDING ED

It is imperative to understand that not all erectile dysfunction problems stem from psychological issues. There may be an underlying medical cause in patients with erectile dysfunction. For example, a man married a woman and later they found out that he is suffering from erectile dysfunction. Concerned and scared, the woman urges the man to seek medical attention. But because of shame and embarrassment to be known that he has an erectile dysfunction problem at such a young age, he did not go to the doctor. Later, he was soon suffering from other symptoms that he did not think relates to erectile dysfunction. The woman persisted to tell him to visit his doctor as their sexual relationship is now being affected by the erectile dysfunction. And finally he did. It was soon found through blood tests and other laboratory tests that he has a tumor growing in his pituitary gland, which was causing a deficiency in his testosterone level. His erectile dysfunction was due to that tumor, and as soon as that tumor was removed, he later began to enjoy a full and satisfying sexual relationship with his woman.

So, to clarify what I have written here, I would like to tell the reader that erectile dysfunction is not all in the head. Although sometimes it is because depression, anxiety and stress can affect a man's libido, it is still very important that patients should have his erectile dysfunction checked as there might be an underlying medical condition that might be chronic. With the treatment of this condition, he can gain back his full erection and maintain it to satisfy himself and his partner.

Erectile dysfunction, in most cases, can be treated. It is a problem that should be addressed and not hidden. It is a problem that once treated can boost a man's self esteem, as this suffers the most because man thinks that masculinity is measured by his sexual performance. There are many helpful drugs now circulating in the market that addresses erectile dysfunction. The most popular choice is Generic Viagra, the first brand name erectile dysfunction medication that came out. Others are Levitra, Cialis, Kamagra, and Vimex (an herbal pill). If these medications do not help a man's erectile dysfunction, there are other methods to try like injecting drugs directly into the penis, vacuum devices that enlarges a man's penis and implantable penile prosthesis. If this does not work yet again, microvascular surgery is another option that a man could try for his erectile dysfunction problem as this procedure is performed to reestablish blood flow into the penis. This is usually done for patients with vascular diseases or injuries.

TYPES OF ERECTILE DYSFUNCTION

Erectile dysfunction, also known as impotence is a condition where a man faces the problem with the erection of the penis. Having a problem with erection once in a few months is totally normal. Erectile dysfunction becomes a matter of concern if it's an ongoing problem. Most of us know that erectile dysfunction occurs when the blood vessels in the penis can't expand and receive enough blood. Another dysfunction or problem-related to the penis that many men face is the condition of prolonged erection. It also happens due to abnormality in the blood circulation in the penis.

The abnormal flow of blood to the penis that causes prolonged erection is called priapism. In some cases of priapism, the erection may even last for more than 4 hours. Such a condition is very painful and can happen even without sexual arousal.

1. Low Flow Erectile Dysfunction

It is also known as low flow or ischemic priapism. This type of erectile dysfunction occurs when the blood traps in the spongy tissues called erection chambers of the penis. Mostly, the cause behind ischemic priapism remains unclear. But, according to doctors, men who suffer from sickle cell disease, blood cancer (leukemia) or malaria have increased chances of ischemic priapism effects. Delaying proper treatment for these conditions causing ischemic priapism can result in permanent erectile dysfunction or impotence.

Symptoms of ischemic priapism include the following:

• Increasing penile pain

• Rigidity in the shaft of the penis while the glans remains soft or unhardened

If you face any of the above-mentioned symptoms related to priapism, you must immediately consult a specialist doctor. Proper and timely treatment of priapism is necessary. Otherwise, the following complications can arise

Complications that can arise due to priapism:

Ischemic priapism, if left untreated can lead to serious complications. In ischemic priapism, blood traps in the penis for a prolonged period of time. When this happens, the oxygen levels in the blood start dropping. Due to a lack of enough oxygen, the penile tissues can get damaged. The damage to these sensitive tissues is irreversible and thus it can cause permanent erectile dysfunction or disfigurement of the penis.

In rare cases, priapism can even lead to serious vascular problems in the penis, which in turn, can cause the death of penile tissues (penile gangrene). Therefore, it is wise to seek timely medical help for priapism and save yourself from any unforeseen trouble.

Treatment for Priapism

Depending upon the cause and type of priapism, your doctor will tell you about the treatment option best suited for you. For erections lasting between 4-6 hours, medications can be really effective. These medicines narrow the blood vessels in the region, thereby reducing the blood flow to the penis chambers.

If medicines do not provide relief even after 6 hours other treatment options may be required. These treatments include aspiration and surgery. In aspiration, the doctor numbs the penis using some medications and then drains the accumulated blood with the help of a needle. Aspiration provides quick relief from the pain and swelling. If none of the above treatments works, surgery may be re□uired. In the procedure, the doctors drain out the excess blood and then reroute the blood. This ensures proper blood circulation to the penis.

If in your case, the priapism is recurrent, your doctor will try to evaluate the root cause. Your doctor may prescribe medicines like decongestants which reduce blood flow to the penis. In cases where priapism occurs as a result of sickle cell anemia, leukemia, or other disorders, the underlying condition is treated to ensure that priapisms do not occur again.

Tips To Follow While Dealing With Priapism

Ice packs are soothing– Prolonged erection, of course, becomes painful and discomforting. Thus using an ice pack helps in relieving the pain. You can apply the ice pack on the penis or in the perineal region to subside the swelling. Ice packs are highly beneficial in high flow erectile dysfunction (non-ischemic priapism). If you are apprehensive, then here is assurance for you that there are no side effects of using ice packs for priapism. Usually, doctors also advise the same along with the ongoing treatment to hasten the process of relief.

Alcohol and tobacco can cause permanent damage- If you are already dealing with erectile problems, then alcohol and tobacco are a big no for you! Alcohol and smoking are known to aggravate the condition. Men who have priapism due to sickle cell disease must refrain from consuming these. Alcohol and tobacco are known to act as major triggers for sickle cell crisis. Hence, it can result in permanent erectile dysfunction.

Exercise for symptomatic relief– Mild exercises that improve blood circulation throughout the body is very effective in erectile problems. The most effective physical exercise for priapism is climbing stairs.

Follow these tips and receive the proper treatment to free yourself from this temporary trouble. Stay healthy Stay happy!

2. *High Flow Erectile Dysfunction*

It is also known as high flow or non-ischemic priapism. This condition is rarer in comparison to ischemic erectile dysfunction and causes lesser pain. High flow priapism happens as a result of an injury to the penis or near the scrotum that is severe enough to cause a blood vessel to rupture. This rupturing of the blood vessel disturbs the normal blood flow in the penis.

- An erection that lasts for more than four hours even without sexual stimulation

- The shaft of the penis is not completely rigid during erection

SYMPTOMS OF ED

Normal male sexual function generally starts with sexual desire or libido involving the stimulation of the brain, nerves, blood vessels and hormones, and the erection of the penis by becoming firm, the release of semen (ejaculation) and ends finally with having an orgasm. An erection is achieved when the muscles of a set of spongy tissues in the penis, namely the corpora cavernosa, relaxes to allow the inflow of blood into the spongy tissues resulting in the expansion and firmness of the penis. To sustain this erection, another set of muscles blocks the outflow of blood once an erection is achieved. When there is a disruption or impairment of any or more of these processes involved in achieving an erection as a result of several psychological, neurological, hormonal or vascular causes, this will lead to the inability of the man to achieve or maintain an erection that is sufficient for satisfactory sexual activity. This situation is what is generally referred to as male Impotency or Erectile Dysfunction(ED).

ED is relatively a common problem affecting over 150 million men worldwide. However, according to The Mayo Clinic, "an occasional episode of Erectile Dysfunction is normal" but then states that "When erectile dysfunction proves to be a pattern or a persistent problem, however, it can interfere with a man's self-image as well as his sexual life. It may also be a sign of a physical or emotional problem that re□uires treatment." Therefore, failure to achieve an erection less than 20 percent of the time is not unusual, and may not re□uire any treatment. It is the failure to achieve an erection more than 50 percent of the time, which should generally be indicative of a problem and therefore re□uiring treatment.

Erectile dysfunction is one such problem for males that can make their personal life frustrating. It is the inability of a male to maintain the erection of the penis. This affects the sex life of both partners. This condition can be really disappointing and may cause emotional turbulence in the person as well. Although effective treatments for erectile dysfunction are available, most men hesitate to talk about it with anyone. So, many men who face the issue of erectile dysfunction choose to suffer in silence. But, choosing your health over hesitation is the only wise decision. Early detection of erectile dysfunction can save you from dealing with serious complications. There are certain symptoms of erectile dysfunction that you should look out for as warning signs.

This is one of the most common and early signs of erectile dysfunction. Usually, there can be much difficulty in retaining the erection for sexual intercourse. Although, it is not true that you will never achieve an erection, the chances of easily erecting the penis decrease majorly. There is a huge possibility that even if you manage to make the penis erect, it won't be rigid (softer than normal erection). If it happens frequently with you, then it is a clear sign that you should get in touch with a specialist to determine the underlying cause.

Reduced Sex-Drive (Libido)

Fairly low sexual desires and a reduced interest in sexual activities is another major sign indicating erectile dysfunction. There are chances that reduced sex-drive can be due to other physical and psychological factors as well.

The common psychological factors that affect your interest in sex are stress, anxiety, and depression. Most of the time, it is a clear sign of erectile dysfunction if the above-mentioned symptom also appears simultaneously. So, it is obviously better to discuss your condition with a doctor when it starts bothering you. The more you delay seeking help, there are more chances that your libido may get adversely affected.

Penis Sensitivity Reduction

Your penis has to be sensitive enough for sexual arousal. The reduced sensitivity of your penis can prevent its erection.

Factors that reduce the sensitivity of the penis are:

- *Tight Foreskin*

    The foreskin of the penis becomes very tight. It becomes really difficult to retract it over the glans penis. This medical condition is called Phimosis. Phimosis definitely affects the overall sensitivity of the penis. It also makes sexual intercourse painful and uncomfortable for males.

- *Injury of The Penis*

Injury to the penis has high chances of creating complications in achieving an erection. The injury can be the result of any athletic/sports activity or even rough coitus.

- *Urinary Infection*

Urinary infections affect the health of the penis. UTIs not only cause a problem in passing urine but also in achieving erection and ejaculation. As UTIs have effective treatments that are easily available, erectile dysfunction resulting from this can be easily treated.

Unusual bending of the penis during erection

This abnormal condition is called Peyronie's disease. In other words, it is also known as the 'curvature of the penis'. This is a very rare condition that causes erectile dysfunction. You cannot take this symptom of erectile dysfunction casually as the abnormal bending causes much pain. In Peyronie's disease, scar tissues start getting accumulating under the skin of the penis. This unusual growth of scar tissues causes the penis to bend while erection. You should immediately seek medical consultation if you ever face this condition.

Premature ejaculation

It is a very common symptom found in men dealing with erectile dysfunction. As soon as the ejaculation happens, the penis loses its erection and turns softer. It is quite a common problem that interferes with the sexual life of males.

Anorgasmia

This warning sign of erectile dysfunction is not very common. Anorgasmia is a kind of sexual dysfunction in which a man cannot erect his penis even after sufficient stimulus. It can be □uite frustrating for men and needs immediate medical attention.

These are some of the warning signs that you must not ignore and get medical help as soon as possible. There are certain exercises and food that can help you in improving erectile dysfunction. So, bring out the necessary and healthy changes in your lifestyle and diet to keep away from the stressful condition of erectile dysfunction. Make sure that your diet is rich in vitamins (A, B, C, and E), iron, zinc, calcium, and magnesium. Also, if you perform yoga asanas and exercises every day, it will in improving not just your sexual health but your overall mental and physical health.

☐

CAUSES OF ERECTILE DYSFUNCTION

Most of the people consider erectile dysfunction (ED) as a psychological problem. However it is not the case. Although psychological factors are involved in the causation of ED but mostly we do have any underlying physical cause of ED. Causes of Erectile Dysfunction. With regard to the causes of erectile dysfunction listed above, The Mayo Clinic has this to say: "The physical and nonphysical causes of erectile dysfunction commonly interact. For instance, a minor physical problem that slows sexual response may cause anxiety about attaining an erection. Then the anxiety can worsen your erectile dysfunction." So men who are suffering from erectile dysfunction do not need to bear it in shame. It should be understood that most men will experience this and that there are ways and methods to cure and treat erectile dysfunction. Gone are the days when men are ignorant and refuse to seek help for their problem. As I would like to say, if you want sex that bad but cannot, then go get something done for it.

For most men the causes of ED can be due to a psychological, neurogenic, vascular or drug-induced factor, or a combination of these factors.

1. *Physical Conditions Leading To ED*

1. *Diabetes*

Males suffering from diabetes mellitus usually experience erectile dysfunction at some point of life particularly when they don't have an optimum sugar control. The erectile dysfunction associated with diabetes is attributed to damage to blood vessels as well as nerves.

There are some lifestyle choices which can increase the risk of erectile dysfunction. They include smoking, drinking, and drug abuse. The do so by interfering with the blood supply of the penis.

Trauma to the blood vessels and nerve supplying the penis can also cause erectile dysfunction. The importance of trauma as a cause of erectile dysfunction has been implicated in people who have been riding bicycle for longer period of times. This is because bicycle seat can put constant pressure on the vessels and nerves supplying the penis thereby damaging them and resulting in erectile dysfunction.

4. Medications

There are certain drugs that can cause erectile dysfunction. They include medications used to lower blood pressure and also some antidepressant. The irony is depression and high blood pressure are some of the causes of erectile dysfunction and the drugs you are using to treat these conditions also cause erectile dysfunction. This is why it is important for you to talk to you doctor if you are on any medications and you start having problems with the erection.

5. Surgery

Mostly older people above the age of 50 have problems with erection. This is the age when people also present with enlargement of the prostate and even with prostate cancer. They re□uire surgeries for these conditions and during surgery the nerves supplying the penis might be damaged resulting in erectile dysfunction.

2. Psychiatric Conditions Leading to ED

The brain is involved in achieving erection as well as pleasure and excitement associated with sex so any problem that interferes with functioning of brain can cause ED. Psychiatric conditions are responsible for only about 10-15%of the cases of ED. They include

- Stress

- Anxiety

- Depression

- Low-self esteem

3. Psychological Causes Of ED

This accounts for about 15-20% of most reported cases of ED. Common causes of Psychological or 'Psychogenic' erectile dysfunction include performance anxiety, work stress, and strained personal relationships or reduced attraction for his partner (which may not be associated with a relationship problem). Also, past sexual trauma, misconceptions about normal sexual functions, childhood sex abuse, and suppressed feelings about sexuality are possible causes of psychogenic erectile dysfunction.

4. Neurogenic Erectile Dysfunction

If there is a possible physical problem with the nervous system, this can lead to to the development of ED. The male erection system depends on an intact nervous system to function; therefore any injury to the nervous system involved in erections may cause erectile dysfunction.

Diseases such as Parkinson's disease, Alzheimer's disease, stroke, or head injury can lead to erectile dysfunction by affecting the libido, or by preventing the initiation of the nerve impulses responsible for erections. Also men with a history of pelvic trauma, pelvic surgery such as radical prostatectomy, cystectomy or colectomy may have injury to the cavernous nerves that control erection. Peripheral neuropathy due to, for example, diabetes or excessive alcohol consumption may also affect some nerves as well as causing erectile dysfunction. This cause of erectile dysfunction accounts for about 10% to 15% of cases.

5. Endocrinologic/Hormonal Causes of ED

Diseases and conditions which decreases the level of circulating testosterone in the body, such as castration or hormonal therapy used to treat prostate cancer, will decrease libido and impair erections. Androgen and prolactin levels are of particular concern here as a high level of circulating prolactin causes inhibition of gonadotrophin releasing hormone which lowers the level of testosterone.

6. Vascular Causes of ED

High blood pressure, diabetes mellitus, hypertension and hyperlipidaemia are underlying causative factors for vascular impairment. These conditions lead to the partial or complete loss of the ability to not only achieve but also maintain an erection long enough for it to be useful to its owner and his partner. Also, high triglyceride and cholesterol, pelvic irradiation treatment of prostate, bladder and rectal cancers may damage blood vessels to the penis over time.

Drugs and Erectile Dysfunction

The usage of street drugs such cannabis, cocaine, amphetamines, and heroin can lead to decreased erectile function. Also certain anti-depressants or anti-psychotics have been associated with erectile dysfunction, especially those drugs that regulate serotonin, noradrenaline and dopamine. Excess alcohol intake has also been acknowledged to affect ED.

Medicinal Cause of Erectile Dysfunction

Erectile dysfunction (ED) is a common identified sexual health-related problem that millions of men around the world face. It is a condition where a man is not able to keep with the erection of the penis. There are various factors that contribute to frequent episodes of erectile dysfunction. Lifestyle, dietary habits, and the medications you take play a crucial role in the erectile issues. Facing dysfunction with erection once in a few months is fine, but when the frequency increases or ED becomes regular, it is a matter of worry.

Here we will tell about the medicines that can cause erectile dysfunction. That's not it, there are some simple yet amazing tips further also. So, let's fill you in with all the necessary information for your well being.

Medicines that can trigger episodes of erectile dysfunction are as follows:

1. Antidepressants

Antidepressants usually work by increasing the amount of serotonin in the brain, which makes them feel less anxious. However, high amounts of serotonin can lead to reduced libido and thus create problems while achieving and maintaining erections. Excessive serotonin can also reduce dopamine levels and make the sexual arousal more difficult, eventually leading to erectile dysfunction.

2. Antihistamines

It might come as a shock to you, but certain medicines used to treat allergies can also interfere with your sexual life. Antihistamines like Ranitidine, Promethazine, Hydroxyzine etc. are very commonly associated with erectile dysfunction episodes in men. This happens because of antihistamines block the action of a chemical compound called histamine. This chemical is involved in allergic reactions but in addition to this, histamine is also required for healthy and firm erections.

3. Tranquilizers

Tranquilizers, that are often employed for the treatment of anxiety, insomnia, and muscle spasms, also contribute to erectile problems in men. These drugs have sedative and muscle-relaxant effects which reduce sexual interest and sensation. Tranuqilizers may also interfere with testosterone production, thereby contributing to decreased libido, which in turn causes erectile dysfunction. (Also Read: Can lifestyle and psychological factors cause erectile dysfunction)

4. Diuretics

Diuretics is another class of medicines that can result in erectile dysfunction. Diuretics can hinder proper and healthy erections by reducing the force of blood flow to the penis. Diuretics are also known to deplete zinc levels in the body. Since zinc plays a crucial role in testosterone production, diuretics are often linked with erectile issues.

5. Chemotherapy and Hormonal Medicines

Chemotherapy and hormonal medicines used in the treatment of certain types of cancer can also cause erectile dysfunction in men. Chemotherapy and hormonal medicines often reduce testosterone levels in the body.

This, in turn, results in decreased sexual drive and difficulties in achieving erections. Also, chemotherapy causes a lot of fatigue. This may also contribute to a reduced sexual desire and thus cause problems during erections.

6. Beta-Blockers

Beta-blockers are a type of antiarrhythmic medicines that are prescribed for the treatment of abnormalities with the heart rate and rhythm. One of the very common side effects of taking beta-blockers is sexual dysfunction. This happens because beta-blockers lower the blood pressure. This leads to an insufficient supply of blood to the penis, and thus erectile dysfunction.

Therefore, if you have been facing problems with erections recently and you think that your prescription medicines are interfering with your sex life, discuss the issue with your doctor. Ask your doctors about any alternative medicines and if possible, get your medications switched. If erectile dysfunction in your case is actually due to medications, you will notice significant improvements within 1-2 weeks of switching the medicines.

HOW TO TREAT ED

Occasional erectile dysfunction is a fairly common condition that is often not a cause for concern. Mild stress and other issues can lead to erectile dysfunction from time to time. Frequent and prolonged erectile dysfunction, however, can cause frustration and stress and can impact self-esteem as well. Sexual arousal in males involves the brain, hormones, nerves, emotions, blood vessels and muscles. The cause of erectile dysfunction can be a problem with any of these. Stress and mental health issues also contribute to causing or worsening the condition of erectile dysfunction.

Physical causes for erectile dysfunction include high cholesterol, clogged blood vessels, obesity, diabetes, tobacco use, alcoholism, low testosterone levels, certain prescription medicines, etc. Psychological factors, on the other hand, include depression, stress, poor communication with the sexual partner and other mental health conditions.If a male persistently faces the problem in erecting his penis, it can actually affect his relationship with the partner. It can really be a cause of worry that hinders a male's day to day life. Prolonged erectile dysfunction can also be a sign of an underlying medical condition and is a risk factor for heart diseases.

It is understandable that erectile dysfunction can be difficult for a man to deal with and can cause a lot of frustration and embarrassment. It can also cause insecurity due to the inability to perform sexually. Thankfully, there are a lot of remedies, tips, and treatments that can help you if you are facing erectile dysfunction so that you can lead a healthy sex life. Let's look at some of the tips and remedies that help in improving erectile dysfunction:

 Talk therapy with a doctor

Talk therapy can be very effective in cases where stress and anxiety lead to erectile dysfunction. Your counselor or therapist will talk to you about your feelings about sex or any subconscious conflicts that may be affecting your sexual life. The therapist will then teach you how to reduce your anxiety. The therapist may also ask you to bring your partner along so that they can learn how to support you in the process. Therefore, it will also help in rekindling the emotional bond with your partner.

2. *Exercise improves erectile dysfunction*

Regular exercise can have a great impact and can help in combating erectile dysfunction. Exercises can also include Kegel exercises that focus on improving the strength of the pelvic muscles. Kegel exercises boost the blood flow to the penis, thus increasing the chances of successful erection. A small study conducted in 2005 showed that men who did pelvic exercises regularly regained their normal penile functioning faster than men who did not exercise. Aerobics, swimming, and running also have major effects in boosting the blood flow to the penis. So, ditch the inactive lifestyle and embrace a healthier one to keep away erectile dysfunction

3.   *Yoga can cure erectile dysfunction*

Yoga not just improves the physical but also the psychological causes of erectile dysfunction. Hence, yoga is highly efficacious in cases of erectile dysfunction. Yoga helps in relaxing the mind and body. It also improves the flow of blood to different parts of the body. Yoga is definitely the best natural way to improve erectile dysfunction that is especially because of stress and anxiety.

4.   *Quiting smoking*

In cases where erectile dysfunction is a result of vascular diseases, stopping smoking can be a remedy. Smoking causes narrowing of the arteries. This causes restricted blood flow to the penis leading to erectile dysfunction.

5.   *Healthy diet to beat erectile dysfunction*

Your diet actually plays a crucial role in maintaining your sexual health as well. Diet choices have a direct impact on the problem of erectile dysfunction. Healthy foods like fruits, veggies, fish, whole grains etc. can help in reducing the risks of erectile dysfunction. A healthy diet also helps in maintaining healthy body weight. Studies show that a man with 42-inch waistline (obese) is twice at risk of developing erectile dysfunction than a man with a 32-inch waistline (normal body weight).

6. *Proper sleep schedule to maintain hormonal balance*

Poor sleep patterns can contribute to the development of erectile dysfunction. This is because testosterone levels are proportional to the number of healthy sleep hours. Poor sleep leads to reduced testosterone levels which is one of the major causes of erectile dysfunction.

7. *Limit the intake of alcohol to get rid of erectile dysfunction*

Alcohol can cause temporary as well as long-term erectile dysfunction. This is because alcohol hinders the proper functioning of the central nervous system. This leads to a restricted release of nitric oxide, which is an essential chemical for erections.

8. Acupuncture helps in erectile dysfunction

Acupuncture is a Chinese technique in which needles are inserted at certain points in the body, known as acupoints. Acupuncture works through nerve stimulation and is believed to be quite effective in the treatment of erectile dysfunction.

9. Lifestyle changes

There are certain life style changes which can help in the improvement of sexual function. They include cessation of smoking, exercise and weight loss.

10.   Medications

There is this famous drug called sildenafil which is well known as Viagra. It is not the only drug, rather there is a whole class of drugs called phosphodiestrase inhibitors. The other important medications included in this group are Vardenafil (Levita, Stxyn), Tadalafil (Cialis) and Avanafil (Stendra)

11. Vacuum Pumps

They are specialized devices containing a cylinder and a pump. The penis is placed in the cylinder and pump is used to draw the air out of the pump creating a cylinder. This increases the blood flow to the penis. In order to maintain the erection an elastic band is worn around the base of penis.

12.Surgery

If the erectile dysfunction is due to blockage of the artery supplying the penis especially in younger patients, we can surgically restore that blood flow. The other things we can do surgically is place an implant in there. This implant is filled with the pressurized fluid whenever erection is required.

Erectile dysfunction is a complex problem to deal with. Therefore it is important for you to realize that you have to involve your partner and talk to a doctor if you want to get out of this troublesome situation. The other important issue to keep in mind is to avoid any self-medication at all as it might have lethal outcome.

ED is often a symptom, not a condition. An erection is a result of complex multisystem processes in a man's body. Sexual arousal involves interaction between your:

- Body

- Nervous system

- Muscles

- Hormones

- Emotions

A condition like diabetes or stress can affect these parts and functions and can cause ED. Research shows that ED is mostly due to problems with the blood vessels. In fact, pla□ue buildup in the arteries causes ED in about 40 percent of men over 50 years old.

Your doctor can help identify the underlying cause and prescribe the appropriate treatment. Treating an underlying condition is the first step to treating your ED.

Treatments your doctor may prescribe if your ED persists include:

- Prescription medicine or injections
- Penis suppository
- Testosterone replacement
- A penis pump (vacuum erection device)
- A penile implant
- Blood vessel surgery

- Find roman ed medication online.

- Lifestyle treatments include:

- Sexual anxiety counseling

- Psychological counseling

- Maintaining a healthy weight

- Reducing tobacco and alcohol use

NATURAL TREATMENT FOR ERECTILE DYSFUNCTION

Erectile dysfunction in men is a real threat to men's normal life. It can make you and your lover feeling discouraged and frustrated. This has destroyed many relationships and unions. However, it is not the end of the world as it can be treated and the problem completely solved with natural remedies and disciplines lifestyles that are not difficult to do.

Take the following steps and remedies to treat erectile dysfunction and get your sex life active again:

1. Eat balanced diets

In the one of Dr. Mucher sayings, it states that "the foods you eat have a direct effect on your erectile dysfunction". You must ensure you always eat balanced diets if not for anything but for your condition. Always eat the diets rich in veggies, fish, fruits, whole grains with a little serving of refined grains and red meat. This diet decreases the risk and also helps in controlling erectile dysfunction. Eating balanced diet also assists in keeping a healthy body weight because obesity has been found to aid the potential for diabetes and vascular disease which are agents of erectile dysfunction (ED).

2. Stop smoking

The vascular disease has been attributed to one of the causes of erectile dysfunction. This is so when the supply of blood to the penis is restricted due to narrowing or blockage of the arteries. Blockage of important blood vessels can be as a result of smoking, and this has its adverse effect on firm erection. If you are smoking, take a giant step of stopping it to get the sexual gun back on track.

3. Regular exercise

Exercise is one of the various lifestyles that solve the problem of erectile dysfunction with great result. Studies have shown that exercise plays a vital role in combating progress of erectile dysfunction (ED) and as well as treat it once it has become an issue in your body. A simple brisk walk for 45 minutes help to boost sexual function

4. Have adequate rest

In one of the 2011 Brain Research publishes, one study showed the effect of poor sleep on men's testosterone levels. It confirms that low sex hormones concentrations are attributed to sexual dysfunction. This hormone secretion is researched to regulate the internal lock of the body, and certain hormones are being released with the help of body based on sleep pattern quality. Adequate sleeps and sticking to a good sleep pattern will help your body to release the needed sex hormones to perform optimally.

5. Reduce the alcohol

Both short-term and long-term ED have been associated with alcohol. It was studied that central nervous system is releasing an essential chemical such as nitric oxide which is responsible for aiding and producing an erection, and central nervous system is being depressed by alcohol consumption; thereby reducing its effectiveness. This only implies that insufficient nitric oxide leads to sexual dysfunction.

6. Use Vajiikarana Therapy for Diabetes

Ayurveda recommends Vajikarana therapy for men to improve their sexual function, prevent premature ejaculation, enhance sperm count, boost sperm motility and increase stamina. Ayurvedic doctors recommend

Diabetic Vajikarana Therapy for men who have diabetes. This therapy helps to improve erectile dysfunction in diabetes. Herbs in these preparations help to maintain blood sugar level and also prevent inflammation of reproductive tissues which occurs in diabetes.

7. Try Acupuncture

Acupuncture has turned out to be a new treatment for health issues such as depression, back pain, and as well as erectile dysfunction. Though there have been mixed studies concerning the efficiency of acupuncture for ED treatment, however, there have been positive results and reviews about its effectiveness. A Journal of Alternative and Complementary Medicine publish states that men with erectile dysfunction of antidepressant side effect can benefit from acupuncture. Another study also confirms that acupuncture has been found to help the quality of

erection and improve sexual activity based on about 39%
participants.

8. Take some herbs

Some herbs have been suggested through evidence to
treat (ED) and improve erection by increasing the blood
flow to the penis to improve sexual urge. Some of these
herbs are Ashwagandha, safed musli, Kapikacchu,
Makhana, and as well as fruits like watermelon, mango,
raisins, grapes etc. Use various home remedies to control
diabetes.

9. Ambrina

Your sex life can be a bit of a drag when you are past your
prime. But do not get frustrated about it. It is only
natural. Well, that is if you still have not heard of
Ambrina. Dubbed by critics as a high intensity male
erectile dysfunction remedy, Ambrina is made from

selected natural ingredients. It works like magic in bringing back your long lost mojo in bed. Compared to other herbal supplements, Ambrina poses no dangerous health risk because it is made from the finest herb that possesses natural male enhancement properties.

Manufactured in tonic form, this superb male enhancement remedy is packed with the potent essence of the best Himalayan herbs. It is processed using the highest order of discipline based on Ayurvedic principle combined with the latest advancement in science. This means that you can expect nothing less but a rekindled passion in bed not to mention an enhanced libido that will bring back the memory of your glory days.

This all-natural best selling aphrodisiac works fast. In fact, you can feel its almost magical properties take effect on your manhood in just a couple of hours or less after ingestion. But if you think that the effect of Ambrina is just potent in the present tense wait until you feel its revitalizing effect after prolonged use. Yes. Ambrina has a long-term and profound effect on your sexual health. In fact, you are bound to feel younger and better through years of using Ambrina.

With just a tiny pill, you will find out the difference between Ambrina and your old male enhancement supplement. This hard driving male enhancement product is formulated with the choicest herbs that are traditionally used in effectively treating poor erection, premature ejaculation, impotency, lack of confidence in bed, and weakness during a sexual act. It also works in enhancing your sexual drive by boosting your depleting libido and sexual desire. Aside from this, Ambrina is also known to fuel once vigor and sexual health in the long run.

During a sexual interplay, is not it great for a man to hold his ejaculation on a much longer time? With Ambrina, you can actually maintain longer erection and prevent ejaculating prematurely. Unlike other male enhancement products, Ambrina does not diminish a male's sexual stamina. As a matter of fact, continuous use will help increase your playing time in bed like a charging bull in the heather.

Quick Tips To Treat Erectile Dysfunction(Ed)

1. *Stay active.*

   If you are overweight, lose those extra kilos and stay healthy. Obesity is a major factor that can cause or aggravate a lot of sexual health issues.

2. *Perform regular exercise to improve blood circulation throughout the body*

   You can also try some yoga poses that help maintains overall physical and mental health. Doing so will also alleviate your stress and you will be able to cope up fast with erectile problems.

3. *Eat healthily*

   Include more fibrous and mineral-rich foods in your diet. Switch to more green leafy vegetables and boost your testosterone levels. Avoid junk and greasy foods as these can further add to your misery.

4. Get proper and sound sleep and try to manage your anxiety levels.

It is the most neglected thing when we are all caught in the hustle-bustle of life. Do not let the stress and anxiety pile up and create problems for you.

These are some of the tips and remedies that will surely prove to be wonderful in getting rid of erectile dysfunction. Also, you just make sure to be consistent in following these tips so that the trouble ends faster.

HERBAL TREATMENT FOR ED

There are many causes of erectile dysfunction and if yours specifically relates to poor blood flow since a robust blood flow to the pelvic region is essential for strong long lasting erections, there are some herbs that can help to improve blood flow throughout your body including your groin. The following are the top 3 amazing erectile dysfunction herbs that actually work. Since they are not prescription or OTC medications, they are not only inexpensive but also come few to zero side effects.

Treating erectile dysfunction with herbs is definitely an area for you to consider if you're struggling with this issue and the above 3 are the best erectile dysfunction herbs that you can use. However it's important to remember that these herbs are most beneficial if poor blood circulation is the reason for your ED. If your ED is due to another reason, these herbs may not help.

For thousands of years people have turned to herbalism to deal with various health issues as well as their use to simply promote general health and well-being. This is because many herbs contain many healing properties. With the advent of pharmaceuticals, herbalism may have become less popular but more and more people have started turning back to this ancient healing method because not only are various herbs effective but as mentioned earlier they are inexpensive with few side effects.

One of the best and safest ways to treat erectile dysfunction is by using natural herbs. Natural herbs erectile dysfunction treatment are proven effective and don't cause side effects, that's why many are shifting to this type of alternative medication. In other words, if you would like to steer clear of the side effects of prescriptive medicines do try natural herb erectile dysfunction supplements.

There are various herbal plants used in erectile dysfunction treatment for improving sexual performance. Just try to inform your doctor if you decided to use any of the natural herb erectile dysfunction supplements. And also, some herbs can get in the way with medications, so, it is highly advisable to consult health professionals first.

There are at least seven proven natural herb erectile dysfunction treatments which hail from China, Japan, Peru, and other parts of Asia. These herbs are found to contain

With that in mind, an issue that many men deal with is erectile dysfunction or ED and it's causes may be disease, psychological issues, age, etc, and while there are many solutions on the market including prescription medications such as Viagra, it's important to remember that there are also many effective natural methods that can work including using the following herbs.

1. Yohimbe (pausinystalia yohimbe)

Yohimbe is from the family that includes coffee, madder and gardenia and it's the bark extract which is used for natural healing. This age-old African aphrodisiac's use for treating erectile dysfunction naturally dates back thousands of years and the active ingredient in this herb - yohimbine - has actually been approved by the FDA for treating erection difficulties. While this herb is not as popular as Viagra, it works almost as well and doesn't come with many of the serious side effects associated with the latter, in addition to also treating other health issues that Viagra can't treat such as depression, to help men who have difficulty ejaculating but have no problem having an erection, it can improve women's libido, and so on and so forth. Yohimbe is a bark of a tree and is a well known aphrodisiac to increase libido. It can mostly be found in Africa, this is also being used in parts of Europe as a treatment to impotence. The only set-back is it has side effects that can be serious, even in small doses. Some complaints are nausea, fatigue, dizziness, a severe drop in blood pressure, anxiety, hallucinations, abdominal pain and the worst effect is paralysis. This herb is not allowed to be sold without a prescription.

Yohimbe has been shown by study after study since the late 80s around the world as being able to improve erections which is why it is one of the best erectile dysfunction herbs because its effectiveness has been proven by various researchers. The studies on yohimbe's effectiveness for erectile dysfunction used amounts of 15 to 30 milligrams per day. While this herb can be found easily over the counter, it's best to ask your doctor for a prescription for this herb because what you can get over the counter may only contain very minute amounts of yohimbine which may not make any difference. If you do get a prescription, simply follow the package directions on usage.

Yohimbine comes from the bark of a West African evergreen tree. For the last 70 years, people have used yohimbine as a treatment for ED because it's believed to:

- Activate the penile nerves to release more NO

- Widen the blood vessels to increase blood flow in the penis

- Stimulate the pelvic nerve and boost adrenaline supply

- Increase sexual desire

- Prolong erections

One study found that 14 percent of the group that was treated with yohimbine had full-stimulated erections, 20 percent had some response, and 65 percent had no improvement. Another study found that 16 out of 29 men were able to reach orgasm and ejaculate after completing their treatment.

A combination of yohimbine and L-arginine is shown to significantly improve erectile function in people with ED. L-arginine is an amino acid that helps expand blood vessels. It's regarded as safe and effective for ED but can cause side effects like nausea, diarrhea, and stomach cramps. Avoid taking L-arginine with Viagra, nitrates, or any high blood pressure medications.

In the trials, participants received about 20 milligrams of yohimbine per day, throughout the day.

While tests have shown positive results, yohimbine's adrenaline effects can cause side effects that include:

- Headaches
- Sweating
- Agitation
- Hypertension
- Insomnia

Talk to your doctor before taking yohimbine, especially if you are also taking antidepressants or stimulant medications.

This is from the family which also includes ivy and it's the roots that are used for natural healing. If there was an ultimate herb, it would be ginseng which is why it's sometimes called life root, man root, root of immortality, heal-all, etc.

Ginseng is a natural herb erectile dysfunction supplement that improves over-all wellness and vitality. It is root that helps to loosen artery walls that can lead to smooth flow of blood throughout the body as well as the sexual organs. It is also called a revitalizer. There are two types of ginseng - the Chinese, Japanese or Korean which is p. ginseng, and the American which is p. quinquefolius. While distinctions are made between the effects of the two especially in Eastern medicine, in the West, these two types are generally considered the same.

The reason that ginseng is one of the top erectile dysfunction herbs relates to its ability to dilate the arteries including those that drive blood to the penis. With increased blood flow to the penis, the better your chances for an erection. Several studies have also supported this herb's ability to not only cause an improvement in erection rigidity but also in the penis girth and feelings of arousal which further improve an erection. Men taking ginseng also reported not only firmer erections but also longer lasting erections making ginseng one of the best erectile dysfunction herbs in addition to promoting general health and well-being in every part of the body.

Some of the many healing benefits of ginseng which is why it's called the ultimate "tonic" in the East and an "adaptogen" (i.e. helps the body resist physical and emotional stresses) in the West, include;

- Enhanced immunity

- Improved mental capabilities

- Increased energy

- Increased athleticism

- Improved general well-being, etc

In addition to helping fight diseases and conditions such as,

- Cancer

- Diabetes

- Colds

- High blood pressure

- Male infertility

- Liver damage

- Emphysema

- Increase appetite

- Relive menopausal symptoms

Ginseng has a slight sweet taste and is slightly aromatic and can be used in the form of a powder, tinctures, teas, capsules or tablets which are easily available online and off line. Simply follow package directions on usage. Panax ginseng, a Chinese and Korean herb. Panax ginseng has a 2,000-year history in Chinese and Korean medicine as a tonic for health and longevity. People take the roots of this ginseng, also called Korean red ginseng, for ED as well as:

- Stamina

- Concentration

- Stress

- Overall well-being

Clinical studies show significant improvement in:

- Penile rigidity

- Girth

- Duration of erection

- Improved libido

- Overall satisfaction

P. ginseng works as an antioxidant, releasing nitric oxide (NO) that helps erectile functions. Some people use a P. ginseng cream for premature ejaculation.

Dosage:

In human trials, participants took 900 milligrams of Ginseng 3 times a day for 8 weeks.

This plant is considered a safe treatment, but should be only used on a short-term basis (6 to 8 weeks). The most common side effect is insomnia.

Ginseng can interact negatively with alcohol, caffeine, and some medications. Ask your doctor about how often you can take P. ginseng if you're planning to use it.

3. Ginkgo (ginkgo biloba)

Another popular herb in traditional Chinese medicine besides ginseng in ginkgo which is also popular in India's Ayurvedic medicine and it's the leaves that are used for natural healing. The ginkgo tree is a sacred tree in many parts of Asia and has been used in that part of the world to treat a myriad of health issues for thousands of years. The reason that it's one of the best erectile dysfunction herbs is also the reason that it helps with many of the previously mentioned diseases and conditions i.e. its ability to improve circulation. As mentioned previously, improved blood flow can help to improve erections.

It is commonly used to boost memory and other psychological capabilities because it is said to improve blood flow and oxygen supply to the brain. In this case, it has effect on blood circulation, therefore it helps those with erectile problems. One study found that this herb helped to relieve erectile dysfunction which was caused by the narrowing of the arteries which supply blood to the penis

Ginkgo is usually recommended for the natural treatment of the following conditions,

- Alzheimer's disease as well as MID (multi-infarct dementia)

  - Heart disease

  - Stroke

  - Anxiety

  - Cochlear deafness

- Macular degeneration

- Diabetic neuropathy

- Tinnitus

Using ginkgo for ED

Since it's difficult to get enough of the medicinal properties from using the leaves (to make infusions or tinctures), it's recommended to buy a standardized ginkgo product which contains a concentrated 50:1 extract (50 pounds of ginkgo leaves used to make 1 pound of standardized extract). Follow package directions on usage.

Ginkgo biloba may increase blood flow to the penis. Researchers discovered the effect of gingko on ED when male participants in a memory enhancement study reported improved erections. Another trial saw improvement in sexual function in 76 percent of the men who were on antidepressant medication. This is why researchers believe that ginkgo may be effective for men who are experiencing ED due to medication.

But some studies also report no improvement or differences after taking ginkgo. This may mean that gingko is better for ED management than as a treatment or cure.

Dosage:

In the study where men reported a positive response, the participants took 40 or 60 milligram capsules twice a day for four weeks. They were also on antidepressant medication.

Talk to your doctor if you're considering ginkgo supplements. Your risk for bleeding may increase, especially if you are on blood thinning medications.

4. Maca

A root vegetable from Peru. For overall health benefits, maca is a great addition to your diet. Maca, or Lepidium meyenii, is rich in:

- Amino Acids
- Iodine
- Iron
- Magnesium

There are three types of maca: red, black, and yellow. Black maca also appears to alleviate stress and improve memory. And stress can cause ED.

In animal trials, maca extract significantly improved sexual performance in rats. But this Peruvian root has minimal evidence for its direct ability to improve erectile function. Studies show that eating this root may have a placebo effect. The same researchers also found that maca has no effect on hormones levels.

Men who took 3 grams of maca per day for 8 weeks reported an improvement in sexual desire more often than men who didn't take it. While maca is generally safe, studies do show elevated blood pressure in people with heart conditions who took 0.6 grams of maca per day. It's recommended that your daily consumption be less than 1 gram per kilogram, or 1 gram per 2.2 pounds.

5. Mondia whitei

Mondia whitei, also known as White's ginger, is particularly popular in Uganda, where medicinal plants are more common than medication. It's used to increase libido and manage low sperm count.

Studies suggest that M. whitei may be similar to Viagra in that in increases the following:

- Sexual Desire

- Human Sperm Motility

- Testosterone Levels

In fact, there's even a drink call "Mulondo Wine" that uses M. whitei as an ingredient. M. whitei is considered an aphrodisiac because of evidence that it increases libido, potency, and sexual pleasure. Studies in mice suggest that M. whitei is also fairly low in toxicity.

Other herbs reported to treat ED

These herbs have shown a pro-erectile effect in animals such as rabbits and rats:

- *Horny Goat Weed, Or Epimedium*

- *Musli, Or Chlorophytum Borivilianum*

- *Saffron, Or Crocus Sativus*

HOME REMEDIES FOR ED

1. Boost sexual conflict by putting in more red onion and raw garlic to your food intake. It is suggested to munch one small red onion and three garlic cloves every day. To make it more palatable, try adding it up to salads.

2. Every night before you go to bed, add a few tbsp. of lemon juice and a few tsp. of eucalyptus oil in warm water and have a relaxing bath. Do this every night before retiring.

3. A mixture of honey and avocado is said to rouse sexual desire. Try having this for dinner.

4. Blend parsley, rosemary, and mint altogether and take 1 tsp. every day.

ESSENTIAL OILS FOR ED

Erectile dysfunction, also commonly referred to as impotency, is a very common condition in men. Erectile dysfunction is characterized by the inability of a man to obtain or maintain an erection firm enough for sexual intercourse. Usually, men do not feel comfortable talking about topics like erectile dysfunction. This hesitation and apprehension often lead to delayed treatment. By the time due attention is given to the issue, the condition of erectile dysfunction becomes even worse. Along with the medical treatment of erectile dysfunction, you can also use some essential oils that aid the treatment of erectile dysfunction. Essential oils which usually contain concentrated plant extracts that retain the plant's natural aroma and flavor. Essential oils are usually prepared through mechanical pressing or distillation. Nowadays, owing to the numerous side effects of medications like

Viagra, many men are now shifting towards natural treatment using essential oils.

Essential oils have a number of benefits and can significantly improve the condition of erectile dysfunction.

How To Use Essential Oils For Erectile Dysfunction

When it comes to using essential oils as a remedy for some ailment, topical usage is recommended. However, you should keep in mind that undiluted essential oils should not be applied directly to the skin. Essential oils should be mixed with carrier oils like avocado or almond oils and then used topically. There are a variety of ways in which the essential oils can be applied:

1. Making a hot water compress with the oils and then applying to the kidney, spine or lower back.

2. Mixing the oil with a carrier oil and then massaging.

3. Spraying the oil on your bed sheet

There are various essential oils that you can use to fasten the treatment of erectile dysfunction. Each of these oils have a wide variety of benefits for your physical and mental well-being and can bring about a remarkable improvement in the condition of erectile dysfunction.

1. Ginger Oil

Ginger oil has been used as a natural aphrodisiac for centuries. It is an excellent remedy for erectile dysfunction. It helps improve erectile dysfunction by stimulating the senses of the body and reducing sexual fatigue. Moreover, ginger oil soothes the nervous system, thereby increasing the sexual drive/libido.

2. Cinnamon Oil

Cinnamon oil is yet another old remedial oil to improve reproductive health in males. It boosts the production of testosterone and improves sperm motility. Cinnamon oil also stimulates the nervous system and alleviates the erectile problems.

3. Lavender Oil

Lavender oil has been in use for centuries and has a wide variety of health benefits. For the condition of erectile dysfunction, lavender oil works wonderfully by boosting the blood flow to the penis. Lavender oil smell is even more effective for erectile dysfunction when used in combination with pumpkin pie, according to a study conducted in 2009.

4. Basil Oil

Basil oil is also a strong effective remedy for erectile dysfunction. It is known to improve sperm motility and vitality. Basil oil also reduces oxidative stress in the body. It also helps relieve anxiety so that you can get rid of erectile dysfunction faster.

5. Nutmeg Oil

Nutmeg oil is considered to be one of the most potent oils for improving the condition of erectile dysfunction. This essential oil increases blood circulation in the body and is also a well-known aphrodisiac. It also has a soothing effect on the nervous system and can work quite wonderfully for all your erectile problems.

Rose oil is known for its amazing effects on male sexual health. This essential oil particularly increases the secretion of happy hormones, thereby alleviating stress and anxiety. It also increases the testosterone levels, which, in turn, improve sexual drive.

The above-mentioned oils can be really helpful in hastening the treatment of erectile dysfunction in most mild cases. However, you should understand that these oils alone cannot treat the underlying medical condition causing erectile dysfunction. These oils should be used as a complementary remedy along with proper medical treatment.

Therefore, as soon as you notice the symptoms of erectile dysfunction, consult a specialist doctor, and receive proper treatment. Also, discuss with your doctor which

essential oil you should use for better results.

VITAMINS AND MINERALS GOOD FOR ERECTILE DYSFUNCTION

If you face difficulty in either achieving or maintaining the erection in the penis, you must know that it is erectile dysfunction. Erectile dysfunction is a common issue that millions of men face around the world. Worry not, it is absolutely possible to get rid of erectile dysfunction. All you have to know is that improving the lifestyle and eating habits work tremendously in kicking away the erectile dysfunction. Your diet has to be rich in vitamins and minerals to not just improve your sexual health but also your overall health. And not just foods, you can also rely on some supplements as well. Whatever floats your boat, just make sure that you are consuming nutritious things.

Here are all the vitamins and minerals that are good for erectile dysfunction:

1.   *Vitamin D*

Researches have revealed that there is a very close link between Vitamin D deficiency and erectile dysfunction. According to a US-based study, men with Vitamin D deficiency were at a 32 percent greater risk of erectile dysfunction than men who had sufficient Vitamin D. Therefore, incorporating enough Vitamin D rich foods and supplements in your regular diet can significantly improve the condition of erectile dysfunction. Food rich in Vitamin D- Fatty Fish, Soy milk, Cereals, Cheese, Egg yolks

2.   *Vitamin C*

Vitamin C also plays a crucial role in improving erections. This vitamin increases blood flow and keeps the arteries unclogged, thereby aiding easier erections. In addition to this, Vitamin C also supports the biochemical pathways that lead to the release of nitric oxide, which is essential for achieving and maintaining erections. Thus, if you are dealing with erectile problems, Vitamin C can be of great help to you. Food rich in Vitamin C- Oranges, Lemons, Broccoli, Cantaloupes, Kale, Kiwi

3. *Zinc*

If the root cause of erectile dysfunction in your case is low testosterone levels, zinc can produce some great results. Low testosterone levels lead to a reduced sexual drive, eventually resulting in problems during erections. Zinc plays a major role in boosting the production of testosterone. Thus, zinc-rich foods and zinc supplements can help improve your libido as well as your erections. Food rich in Zinc- Oysters, Chicken, Tofu, Nuts, Lentils, Mushrooms

Recent studies have shown that niacin or Vitamin B3 can work wonders in improving erectile issues. Vitamin B3 is particularly helpful for men with high cholesterol, who otherwise cannot take Viagra and other pills due to their blood-thinning effects. Vitamin B3 supplements, if taken on a regular basis, can bring about significant positive results in moderate as well as severe cases of erectile dysfunction. Food rich in Vitamin B3- Fish, Chicken, Mushroom, Brown Rice, Peanuts, Avocados

5.   *Vitamin B9 (Folic Acid)*

Folic Acid (Vitamin B9) is another vitamin with amazing benefits in the case of erectile dysfunction. Since erectile dysfunction is a part of a vascular issue, improving vascular health can produce good results. Vitamin B9 focuses primarily on this and improves blood circulation throughout the body. Vitamin B9 also acts as a mood stabilizer and thus is effective in the case of stress-induced erectile dysfunction as well. Food rich in Vitamin B9- Dark green leafy vegetables, Beans, Peanuts, Whole Grains, Seafood

6.   *L-arginine*

The amino acid L-arginine has a major role to play in the formation of od nitric oxide, which is necessary for achieving and maintaining erections. Thus, L-arginine foods and supplements can help a great deal in erectile dysfunction caused due to physiological factors. However, L-arginine alone may not work that effectively. A combination of L-arginine and a herbal supplement called pycnogenol is usually recommended for this purpose. Food rich in L-arginine- Chicken, Pumpkin seeds, Soybeans, Peanuts, Dairy

7. *Magnesium*

Magnesium deficiency can be another factor contributing to the development of erectile dysfunction. It aids in the relaxation of blood vessels and allows the penile blood vessels to relax during erections. Low magnesium levels thus can lead to the constriction of blood vessels and impair proper erectile functioning. Therefore, if you are dealing with erection problems, make sure that you take enough magnesium in your regular diet. Food rich in Magnesium- Dark chocolates, Avocados, Nuts, Legumes, Tofu, Seeds, Whole Grains

8. *Vitamin E*

Vitamin E is another great vitamin for erectile dysfunction. It has multiple benefits for the condition of erectile dysfunction. It improves testosterone levels and thus increases the libido. Vitamin E also improves the supply of blood and thus makes sure that enough blood reaches the penis during erections. Therefore, Vitamin E should be an integral part of your diet if you are facing erectile problems. Food rich in Vitamin E- Vegetable oils, Nuts, Seeds, Spinach, Broccoli

Ensuring that your regular diet looks filled with vitamins and minerals will surely bring wonderful results for erectile dysfunction. Well, you should also know that some foods can have a negative impact and may worsen your problem of erectile dysfunction.

Let's shortly tell you the foods that cause or make erectile dysfunction worse:

CLEANSING AND DETOXIFICATION

Cleanse Your Body Naturally with Food

Detox diet vegetables

A healthy diet is the most important way to detoxify. First, remove foods that interfere with detoxification or make you more toxic. Among them include fructose, which is found in soda (as high-fructose corn syrup or HFCS) but also in fruit juices and commercial juice cleanses.

Research shows this simple sugar can become a key contributor to chronic diseases including obesity and ED. A natural cleanse also involves avoiding trans fats and damaged fats. These fats are in processed foods with "partially hydrogenated" in the ingredients — even if the front label says "low in fat." Scrambled eggs on the buffet table are an example of damaged fats, where the fat has become oxidized — skip them.

Foods for Natural Detoxification

1.   Fats and Oils

Natural fats and oils like extra virgin olive oil and organic coconut oil provide energy for the detox and biotransformation processes.

2.   Nuts and Seeds

Try almonds, sunflower seeds, walnuts, and flax seeds for a healthy snack. Nuts and seeds are excellent sources of fiber that assists in proper excretion and elimination.

3.   Proteins

Protein is crucial for the proper function of the two major detoxification pathways inside the liver cells — called the Phase 1 and Phase 2 detoxification pathways. Opt for organic grass-fed beef and wild-caught seafood.

4.   *Legumes*

Beans, lentils, and other legumes are a good source of soluble and insoluble fiber as well as a variety of amino acid precursors.

5.   *Fruits*

Fruits contain a wide variety of phytonutrients, such as beta-carotene, lutein, and anthocyanins that have protective antioxidant properties. They are also a good source of soluble and insoluble fiber and are high in water content.

6.   *Vegetables*

Among their nutrients, non-starchy vegetables provide a wide variety of phytochemicals and fiber.

Essentially, a body-cleanse diet includes plenty of nutrient-dense, lower-sugar, high-fiber plant foods along with excellent sources of protein and healthy dietary fat. It would eliminate most processed foods including inflammatory fats and instead focus on whole, unprocessed, real foods. Food provides nutrients that help your body detoxify, but sometimes providing specific nutrients in therapeutic doses can naturally cleanse your liver and other detoxification organs.

A nutritionally balanced diet can do wonders to your body. It is important to detox the body with a proper cleansing process. During detox process, harmful toxins are released from the body A healthy mind, lean and fit body, and soft and supple skin; almost all of us wish to have these traits. In order to achieve the same, it is imperative to follow a disciplined workout regime with a nutritionally balanced diet. However, before doing all that, it is of utmost importance to detox the body with a proper cleansing process so that harmful toxins are released from the body. Due to tight working schedules, most of us fail to follow various detox programmes. If you wish to detox your body naturally, just a few minor changes in lifestyle could help you to a great extent. We have curated a list of 7 effective tips that are easy-to-follow and also won't take much of your time and effort.

DETOXIFICATION OF THE PENIS

The penis is actually a sensitive tissue composed of blood vessels – veins and arteries, as well as nerves. When a man is having an erection, blood rushes to the blood vessels, making it hard and erect. The corposa cavernosa, the main chamber within the penis where majority of blood circulates, is the main component in penile erection. For a man to maintain a healthy erection, he must make sure that blood circulating to the area is free from blocking substances such as cholesterol and fat. Your diet plays a major role in all of this, so you may need to detox "down there" in order to clean out bad things you've been taking in, increase your blood and boost your stamina. Here's three natural ways to do it

1.   Blackberries

Blackberries are rich in anti-oxidants and fiber. Anti-oxidants help the body get rid of free radicals while fiber flushes toxins out of the body.

Here's a □uick mix:

- ¼ K Blackberries

- 2 Tbsp Grade B Maple Syrup

- 1 L Distilled Water

2.   Beetroot Juice

Beetroot juice is high in NO_3, a nitrate. Nitrates are vasodilators, that is, they open (dilate) the vascular system (blood vessels and capillaries). When your blood vessels open wider, you have increased blood flow throughout the body. Increased and improved blood flow throughout the body confers many health and performance related benefits.

Here's a □uick mix:

- 1/2 of a medium-sized beet
- 1 apple, orange, or pear
- 3 carrots

3.   Probiotics

Probiotics found in natural greek yogurt or just plain natural probiotic pills will do. Another option is Young Coconut Kefir. Drink this delicious probiotic-rich fermented drink and you'll cut sugar cravings, boost your energy and immunity and create younger looking skin to boot! It is an excellent source of potassium and a very good source of natural sodium.

Here's a few honorable mentions:

1. Chamomile – A traditional remedy for stress and anxiety, chamomile acts as a diuretic and nerve tonic.

2. Juniper Berry – Acts as a diuretic, anti-inflamatory, and decongestant. Very useful in helping to regulate blood sugar levels.

3. Ligustrum Berry – Ligustrum Berry nourishes and tones the liver and kidneys and increases blood circulation.

4. Licorice Root – Licorice root fights inflammation and viral, bacterial and parasitic infection. Cleanses the colon, and enhances microcirculation in the gastrointestinal lining.

5. Milk Thistle Seed – Also called Mary Thistle, Milk Thistle protects the liver from toxins and pollutants

by preventing free radical damage and stimulating the production of new liver cells.

6. Turmeric Tuber -Used throughout Southeast Asia and India for thousands of years, Turmeric has been shown to aid circulation, lower cholesterol, and improve blood vessel health. Healers have used Tumeric for years for the treatment of obesity, as it is said to cut the fat from the blood.

Drink Warm Water with Lemon Juice

Start the day with a glass of warm water and freshly squeezed lemon. This wonder combination has the potential to flush out toxins from the body. You may also add grated ginger in the same for better results. Lemon and ginger together improve digestion and give the metabolism a boost. Preparing this drink is an easy task and won't take more than 2-3 minutes. Make sure you are consuming it on an empty stomach for an effective body detox. This is one of the most effective home remedies for body detox.

Swap Caffeinated Drinks with Green Tea

Caffeinated drinks like tea or coffee can do more harm than good to your body. In order to steer clear of its harmful side effects, swap them with green tea, which is a much better alternative. Apart from cleansing the digestive system, it also helps in boosting the body's sexual metabolism, facilitating erectile dysfunction.

Purify Your Body with Water

It is important to keep yourself hydrated at all times. The body needs water to produce saliva, helps with perspiration, and removes waste. Drink enough water in a day; approximately 8-10 glass or 2 litres. Carry a water bottle with you at all times and keep consuming and refilling it as and when you get the opportunity.

Get Adequate Sleep

Apart from detoxifying the body, it is essential to detoxify the mind as well. A full body detox is of utmost importance. A lot of us underestimate the importance of a good night's sleep. Your brain tends to flush out toxins while you sleep as well. Hence, ensure that you are getting sufficient sleep at night.

Now, that we have shared with you a list of effective tips for natural detox, bring them to your rescue and get a healthy mind and body along with soft and supple skin.

NATURAL FOODS THAT WORKS LIKE VIAGRA

Erection problem – or commonly known as erectile dysfunction – is a very serious topic in the medical field. Apparently, it can occur at any age but for various reasons such as diabetes, stress, anxiety, and depression, among many others. Moreover, side effects of certain medicines can also contribute to this issue.

To counter this disturbing problem, people try to use all medications available including Viagra. Although the latter proves to give you a hard-on, it does not increase your libido or desire to have intercourse. So, at the end of the day, you still have erectile dysfunction. Worry no more, though. There are actually foods that can help you win the battle against erection problem. Check them out below!

1. Pine Nuts

Considered as a super food, pine nuts can either be added to various food items or gobbled anytime you want. They have components (zinc being the primary component) that can work up in boosting your desire for sex.

2. Pomegranate Juice

This one here is called the fruit of perfection, and there is an absolute reason why. It is simply perfect for your libido and erectile problem. Thanks to its many antioxidants, this juice can wipe out all free radicals and toxins from your body. More importantly, it is so easy to prepare.

3. Black Chocolate

When doing the deed, it is the cardiovascular system that is working very hard. Hence it is important for you to take care of it. Having a little amount of black chocolate is enough to boost the said system.

4. Bananas

If you want to enhance your sexual performance at a steady rate, then start consuming bananas. They contain an enzyme that is called bromelain (the same enzyme that can be acquired from pineapple). This is capable of increasing the production of sex hormones and boosts your body's energy levels for greater performance.

5. Avocado

Avocado is packed with folic acid that can increase your stamina in bed. Remember that it is rich in vitamin B6, also known has the hormone regulator.

6. Oysters

They are not called love drug for nothing. And believe it or not, oysters were the favorite food of both Cleopatra and Casanova. This one here can boost your dopamine level at a significant rate. It is quite vital for a better testosterone production.

7. Watermelon

Believed to be the new Viagra in town, watermelon releases effects that increase one's libido. Its citrulline amino acid helps improve your cardiovascular system and relaxes your blood vessels.

8. Asparagus

It is among the natural foods in the planet that is high in vitamin B known as folate. It supports in supplying your body's production of histamine. Keep in mind that the latter is very vital for a healthy drive in bed. It is perfect for both men and women.

9. *Maca*

Maca is dubbed as Peru's natural Viagra due to its history in the country's culture. It has been used as a food to increase an individual's strength, energy, fertility, stamina, and libido.

10. *Pumpkin Seeds*

They are rich in zinc same as oysters. This makes them crucial for healthy sperm production in men, as well as preventing the possibility of testosterone deficiency.

11. *Chilies*

Thanks to their ingredient called capsaicin, chilies are capable of accelerating a person's sexual drive. And there is a reason why eating them makes you feel hot. That is due to the chemicals that raise the heart rate and generate the release of endorphins.

12.Garlic

It contains allicin, which produces heat that stirs up the libido. More importantly, it increases the blood flow in the body and thus improves the desire to do the deed.

13.Ginger

Apart from warming your blood, ginger is also proven to improve the blood inflow in sexual organs. So, if you want to work it out tonight, you better sip a cup of ginger tea beforehand.

14.Almonds

If you are looking to resolve fertility issues, then eating almonds is the best way to go. They are rich in zinc and selenium, which are vital for an improved reproductive health.

15.*Coconut Water*

It is worth noting that the human blood significantly consists of electrolytes. Apparently, the latter can also be acquired from coconut water. It does not only improve your blood flow, it also serves as an aphrodisiac.

SAFETY CONCERNS ON ED

- It's essential to take the recommended dosage of treatment only as massive doses can cause psychosis and paralysis.

- Herb should not be taken with ED medications such as Viagra, etc.

- Other side effects may include nervousness, irritability, increased heart rate, increased blood pressure, flushing, tremor, etc.

- ED treatments are not to be given to children and anyone over the age of 65 should start with a small dose and build up gradually if necessary.

- Some people may suffer an allergic reaction.

- If you are on other medications, talk to your doctor before using yohimbe because there may be unpleasant drug/herb interactions.

• Herbs acts as a stimulant which means that some people may become restless, nervous, etc, in much the same way they would if they drank coffee or any other drink that contains caffeine which means that ginseng can lead to over stimulation.

• Some people may be allergic to these treatments.

• Most ED herbs has anti-clotting action so avoid it if you are dealing with clotting issues or taking blood thinners and don't use ginseng two weeks before scheduled surgery.

• Other rare side effects include increased blood pressure, insomnia, heart rhythm disturbance, asthma attacks, breast soreness, etc.

• If you're on other medications, talk to your doctor before using any ED treatments because of possible unpleasant drug/herb interactions.

- Some ED treatments may cause stomach upset, rash, or headache in some people.

- Large doses may lead to irritability, nausea, vomiting and diarrhea.

- Herbs like Ginkgo is usually only given to children to treat dyslexia.

CONCLUSION

In conclsion, erectile dysfunction(ED) is the inability to achieve an erection when sexually aroused, or to maintain an erection long enough for intercourse. Erectile performance can be associated with some things that men have control over. The impact of erectile dysfunction is not limited to men, it extends to their partners as well. Men may feel ashamed and psychologically burdened because of this type of sexual dysfunction. Similarly, women who measure their self-esteem by how well they can incite arousal may be more vulnerable to rejection.

Erectile dysfunction can be caused by innumerable health conditions. A man's nervous system and blood circulatory system work in tandem to help produce an erection. Let's read on how health conditions such as diabetes and heart problems can impair a man's ability to get an erection and maintain it during sex.

Treatment and prevention of erectile dysfunction in men with diabetes do not necessarily need to be through medication as you can effectively treat and prevent this issue with natural means. If you are suffering from or perceiving symptoms of ED and you want to avoid medication means of treatment, there are available means which are natural and just require disciplines or a form of lifestyle changes. All these natural treatments have been discussed above. Follow them vividly, and you will be freed from erectile dysfunction (ED).

Approximately 85% of all erectile dysfunction cases are caused by specific, diagnosable, physical conditions. Most of these problems are treatable, so men facing erectile problems should have a medical check-up. Sometimes impotence can be a risk factor for more serious relationship or emotional issues. Psycho-sexual counselling may help in problem-solving and bridging communication gaps. Good communication is the foundation of any lasting relationship. If your man is suffering from impotence, you can play a major role in helping him to seek proper treatment. You can confront any concerns you may have about erectile problems by telling your partner how much you care about him. Men with impotence tend to withdraw emotionally and physically from their partners.

It is always wiser to first get in touch with a specialist whenever you find yourself dealing with unusual symptoms. So, even if you want to follow a healthy diet and fitness routine to improve erectile dysfunction, still consult a doctor once for better solutions. The doctor will surely give you the best advice and treat the root cause of your problem after proper diagnosis. And, if you feel that there is some underlying medical condition that is causing you erectile dysfunction, feel free to consult a doctor. So, make the wise choice of seeking medical help now and let the hassles go away once and for all.

There is nothing to dread about the treatment of erectile dysfunction. There is no serious surgical treatment for erectile dysfunction. Effective medication is enough to cure erectile dysfunction. So, do not hesitate in seeking medical help as it is the best and safest option to get rid of erectile dysfunction.